Rome and the Secret Box

ISBN: 979-8-9940500-1-9
Printed in the United States of America
First Edition, 2025

Published by

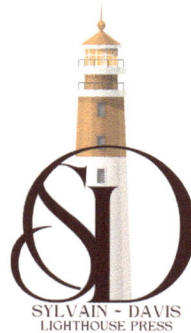

Sylvain–Davis LightHouse Press™

Sylvain–Davis LightHouse Press™ is the official publisher of this work.
All books, educational materials, and digital resources are produced and distributed under the Sylvain-Davis LightHouse Press™ imprint.

Website: sdlighthousepress.com
Email: sdlighthousepress@gmail.com
Instagram: @sdlighthousepress
Facebook: Sylvain-Davis LightHouse Press

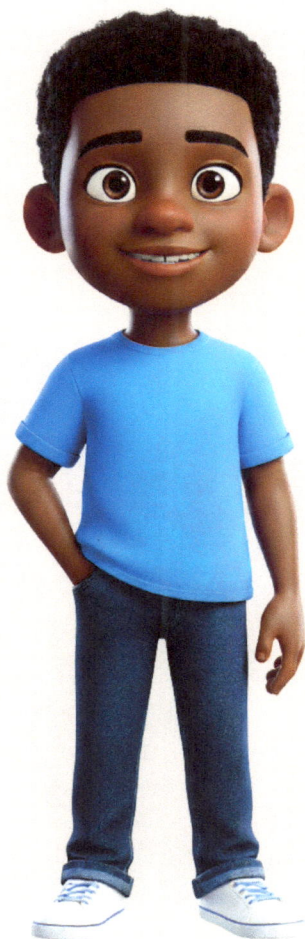

Dedicated to every child who has ever held a secret inside.

May you grow to understand the difference between fun secrets and unsafe secrets, and always feel brave enough to tell a trusted adult when something doesn't feel okay. Your safety will always come first.

Rome loved secrets ~ fun ones, like hiding birthday presents or planning surprises for Mom. He had a shiny gold box for treasures.

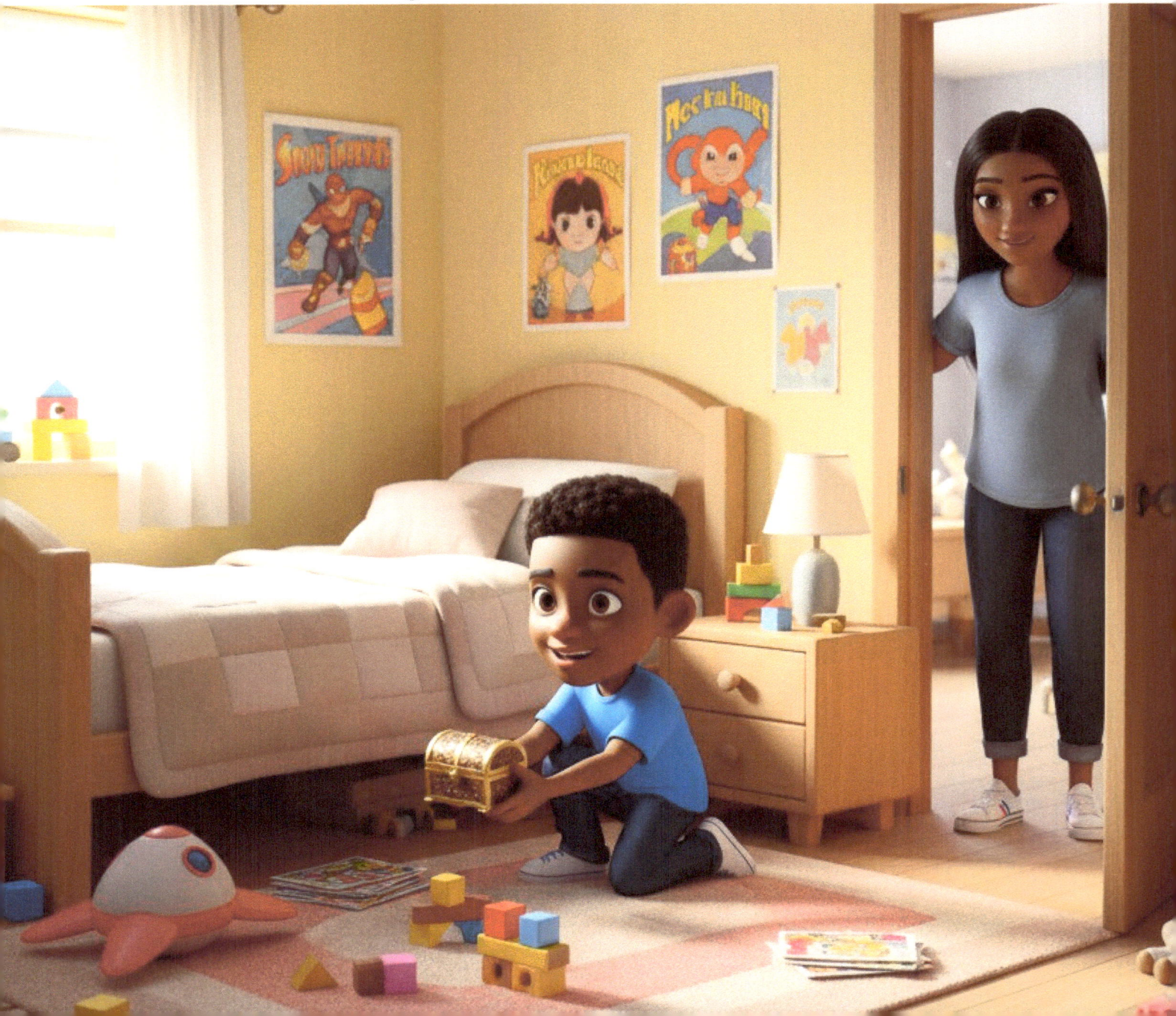

He loved the way secrets made him giggle inside
~ especially when they were happy surprises!

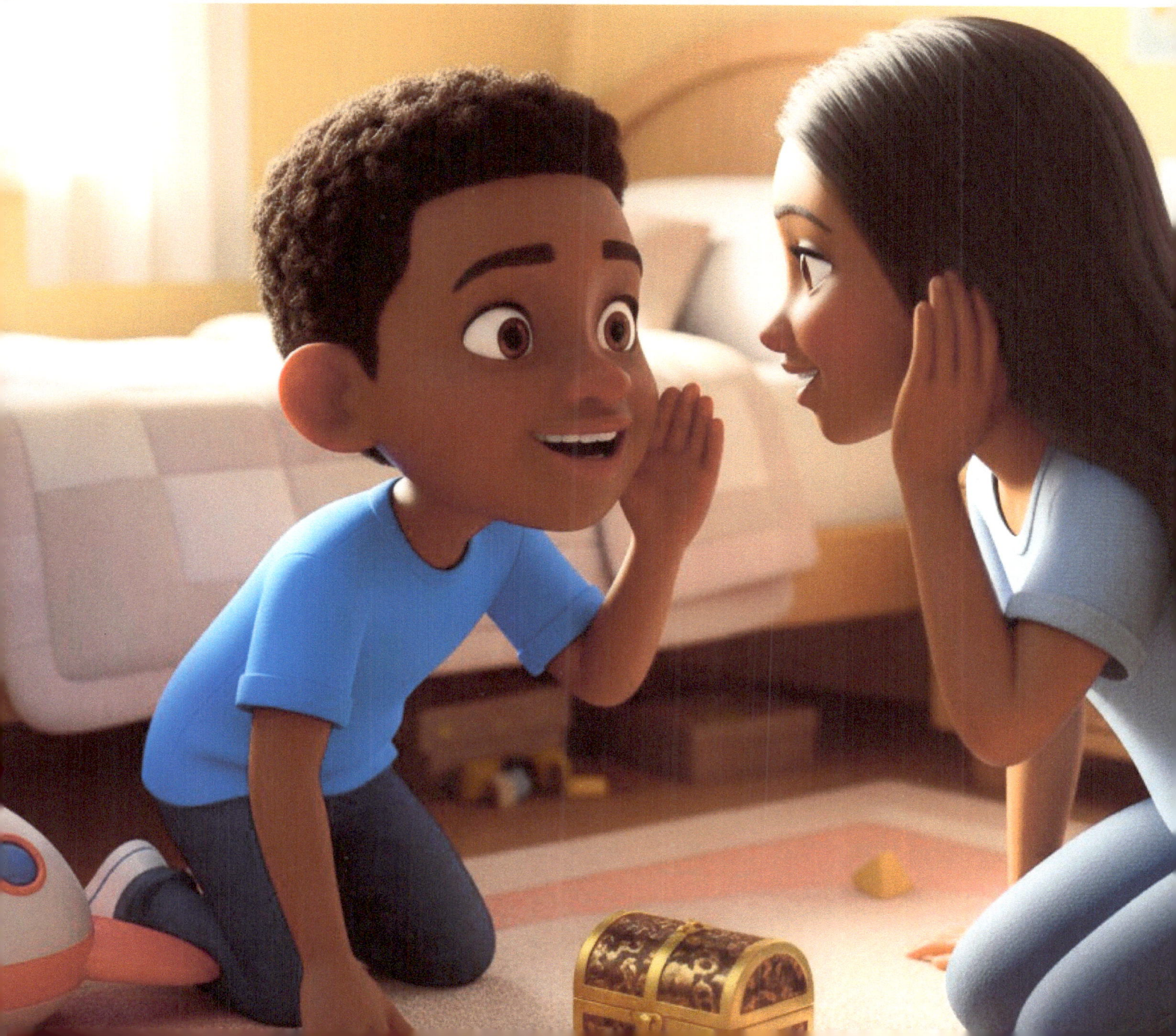

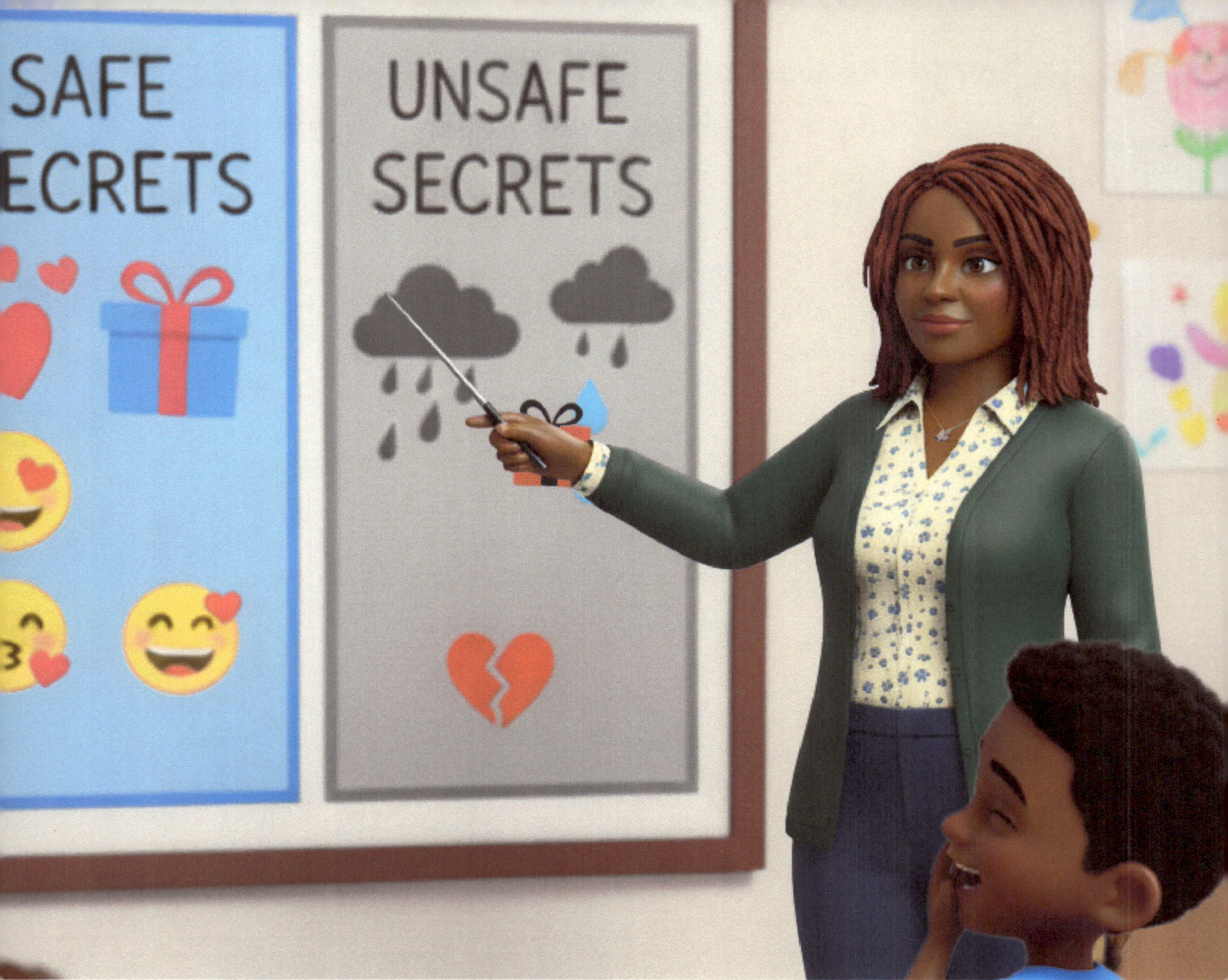

During school, Ms. Teasie taught, "Some secrets are safe... Unsafe secrets make you feel worried or yucky." Rome laughed, "Yucky secrets? Like bad food?"

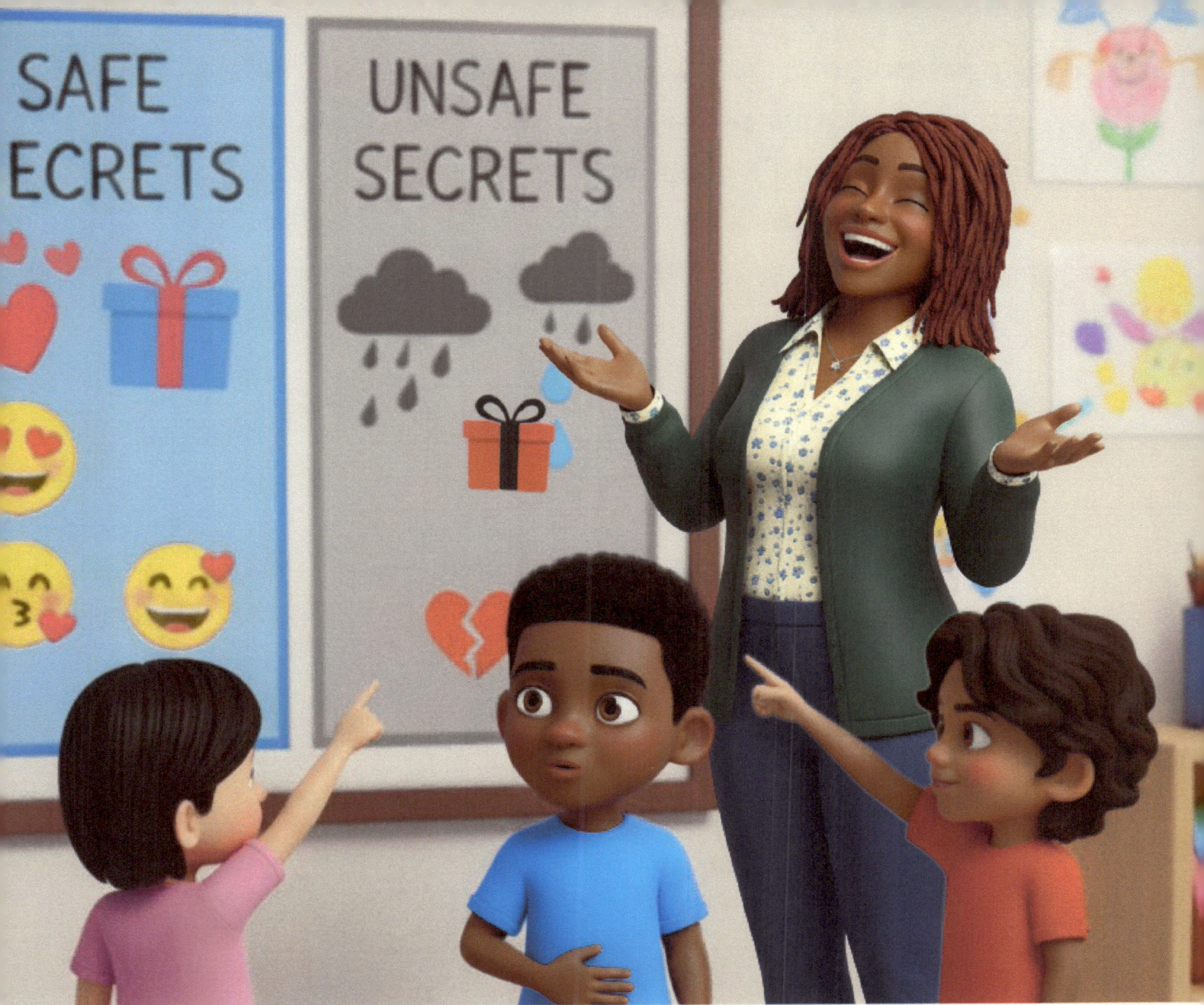

Everyone laughed ~ even Ms. Teasie. "Kind of!" she said. "Safe secrets make you feel happy inside. Unsafe ones make your tummy twist."

After school, Mr. Dan waved from his porch. "Hey, Rome! Want to see my new puppy? But don't tell your mom ~ it'll be our secret!" Rome's stomach felt twisty. He liked puppies, but... Ms. Teasie's words echoed: 'Yucky secrets.'

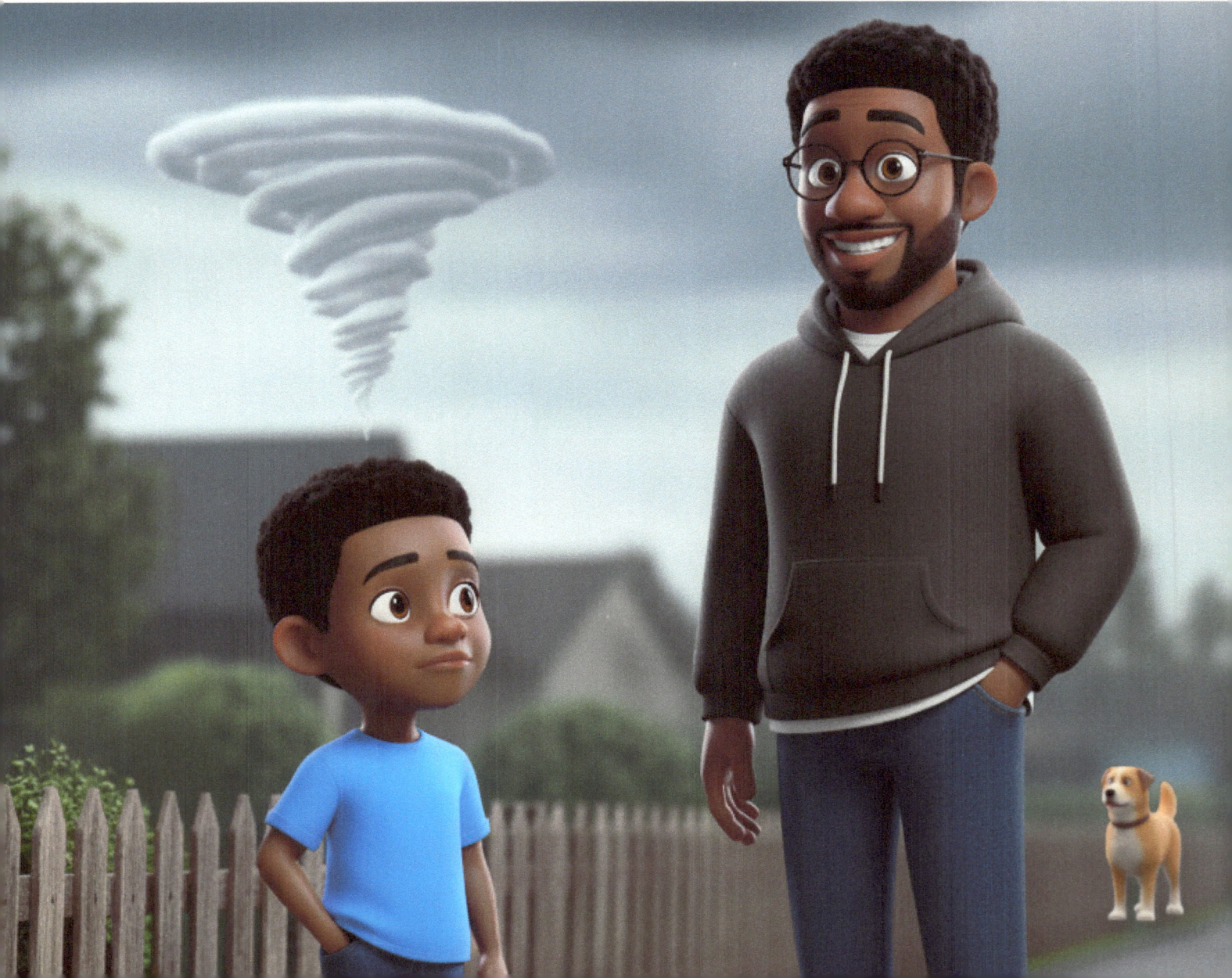

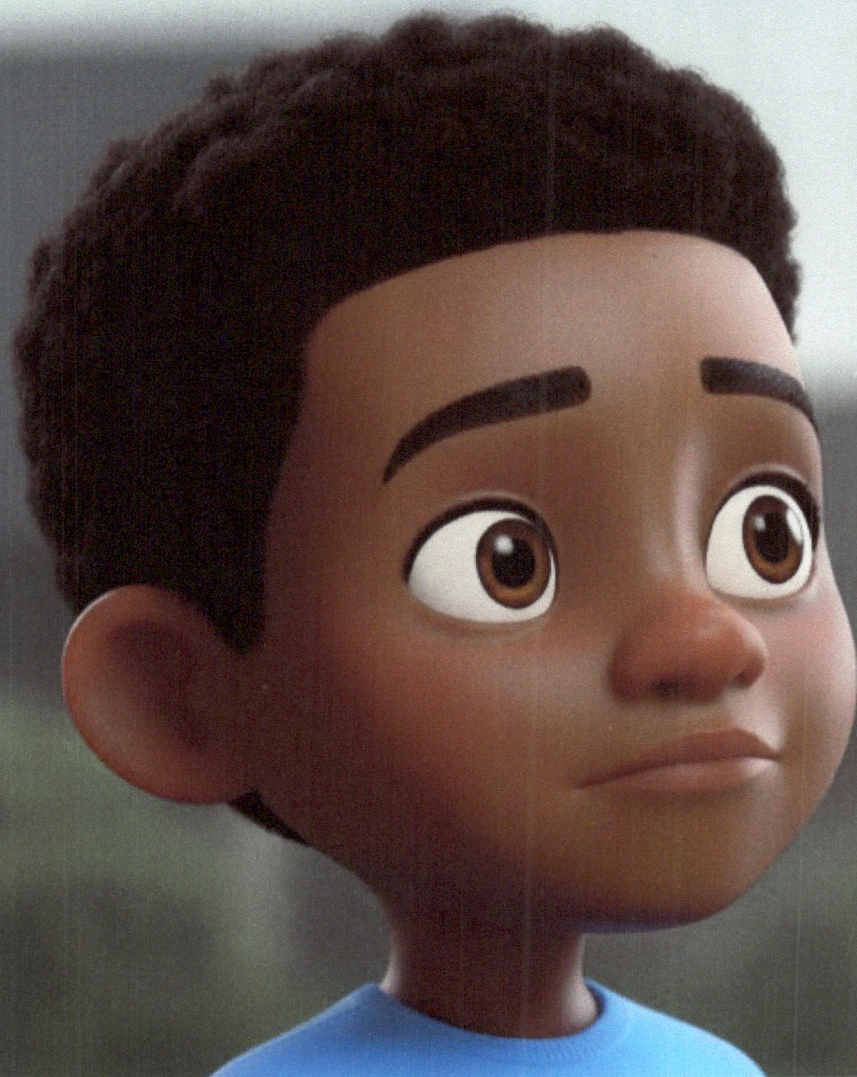

Rome frowned. That twisty feeling again...
maybe this wasn't a good kind of secret.

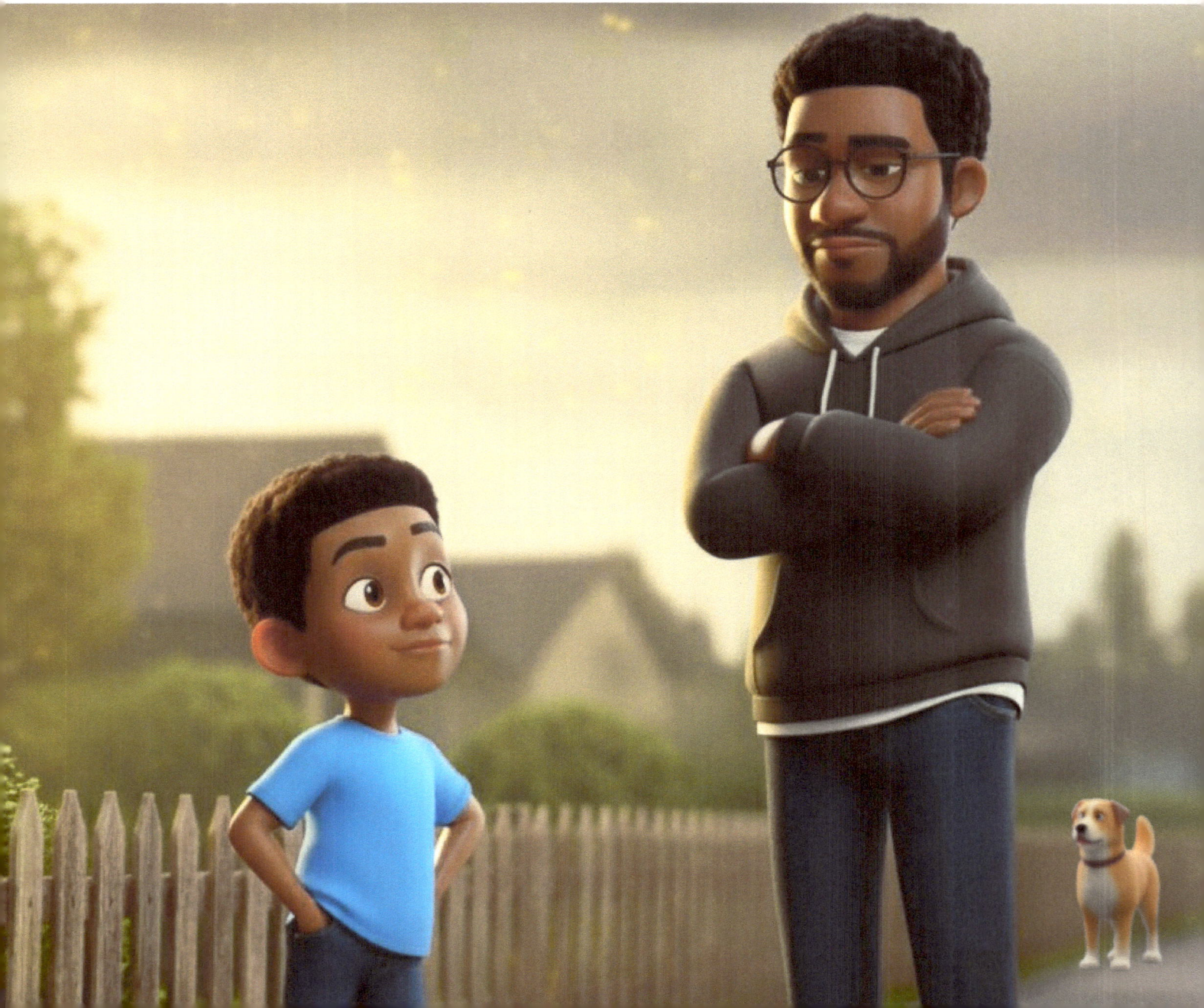

"I can't keep secrets like that, Mr. Dan," said Rome. "My mom says I have to tell her where I'm going."

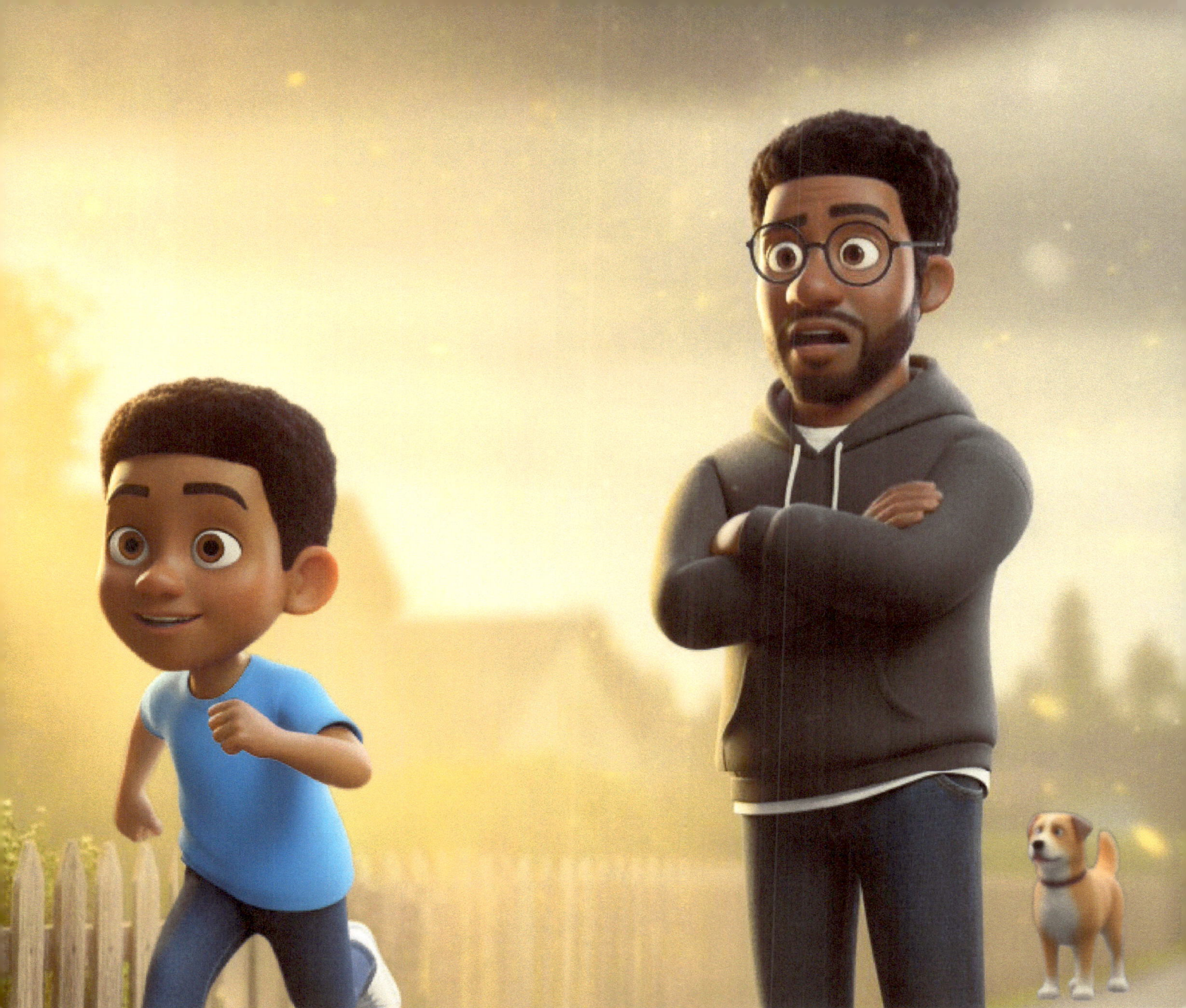

Mr. Dan frowned. "Oh, come on, it's just between us." The twisty feeling came back ~ but Rome knew what it meant. He said louder, "No, thank you!" and ran home.

Rome told Mom everything. He worried she'd be mad ~ but Mom hugged him tight. "I'm proud of you, Rome. You listened to your feelings and told the truth. That's brave."

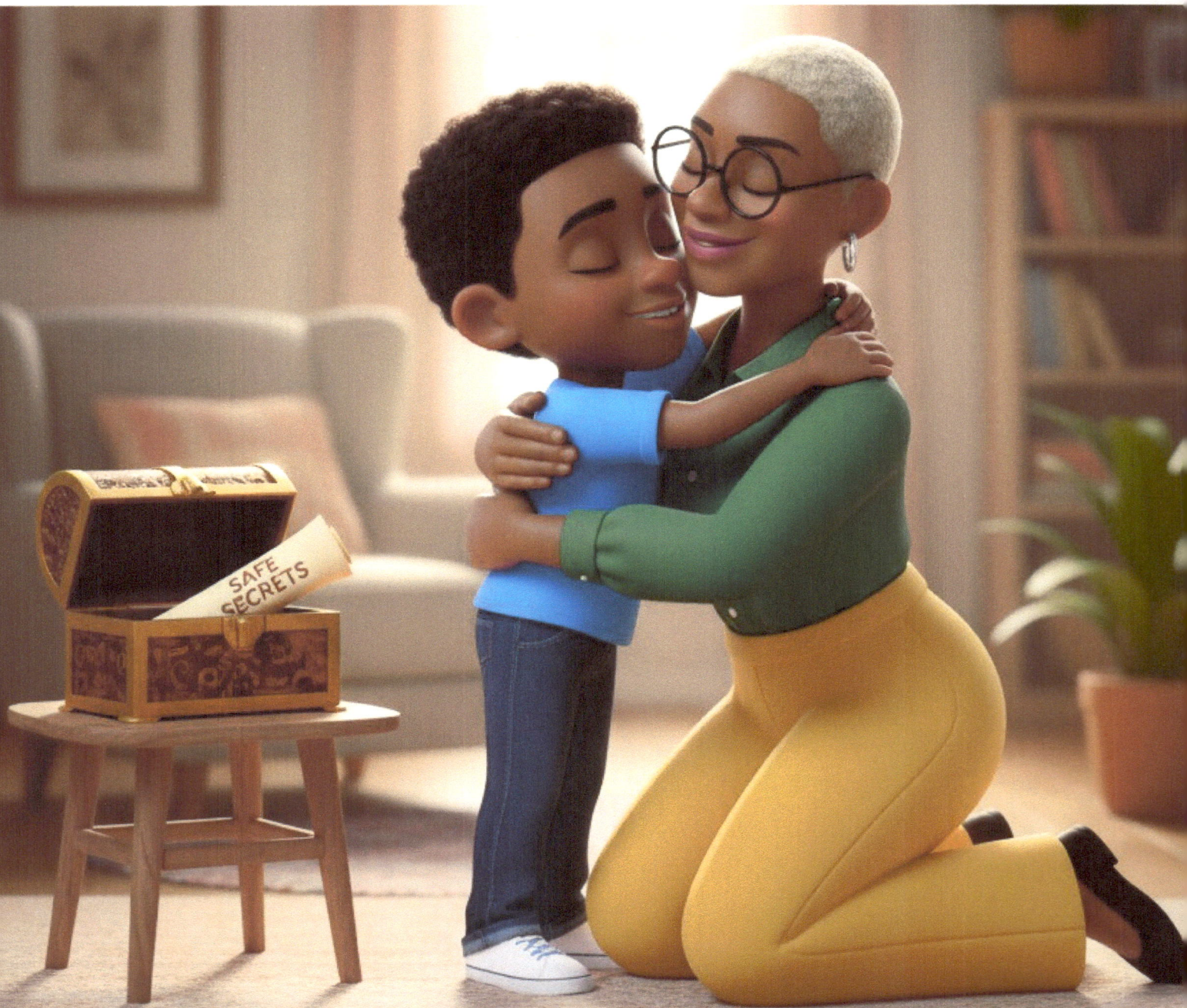

"Safe secrets help people feel good," Mom said.
"Unsafe ones never should be kept."

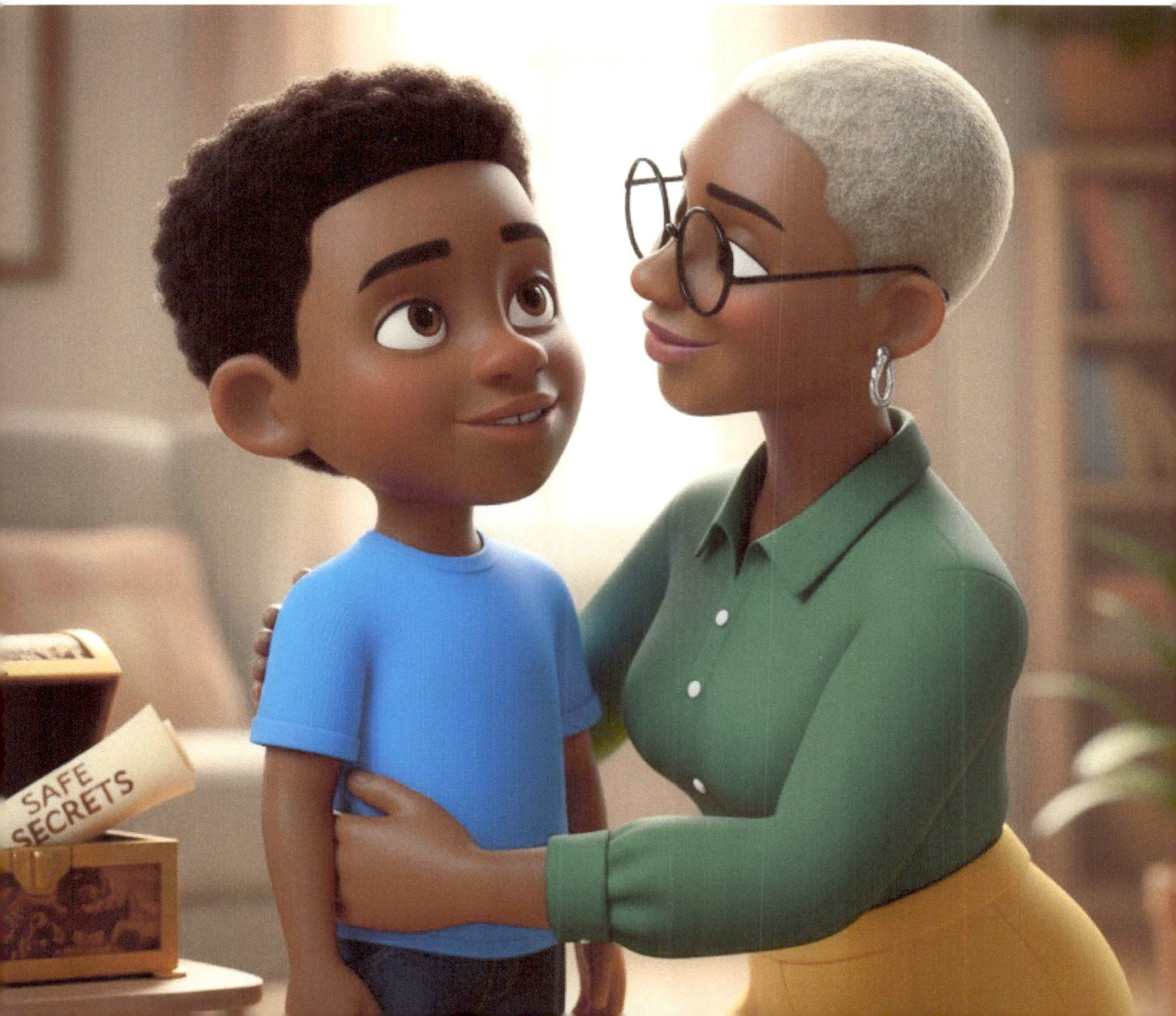

The next day, Ms. Teasie asked, "Who remembers what we do if we have a secret that feels wrong?" Rome raised his hand. "Tell a trusted adult! Keep telling until someone helps!"

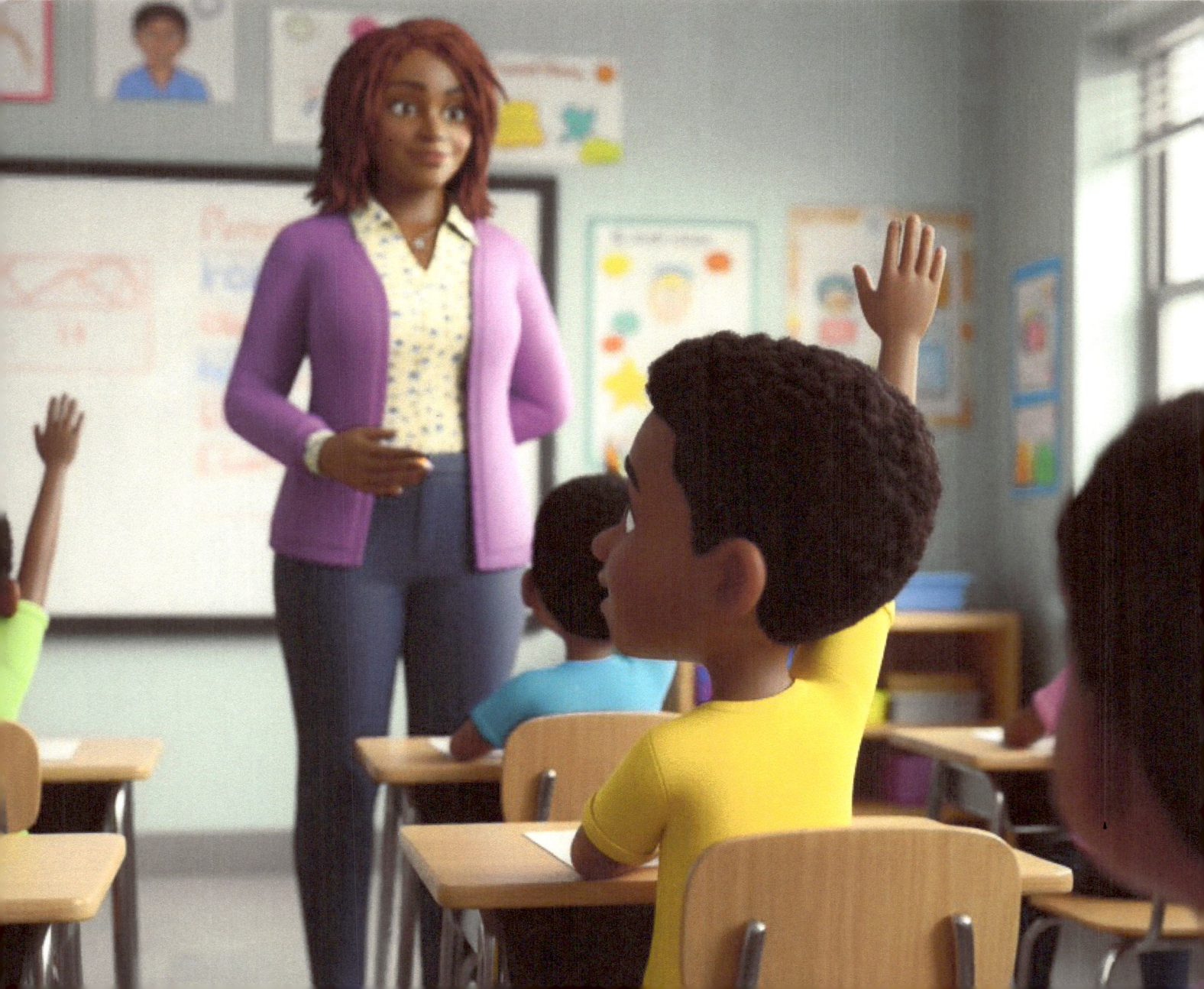

Everyone clapped. Rome smiled ~ his gold box wasn't for bad secrets. It was for drawings and things that made him feel proud.

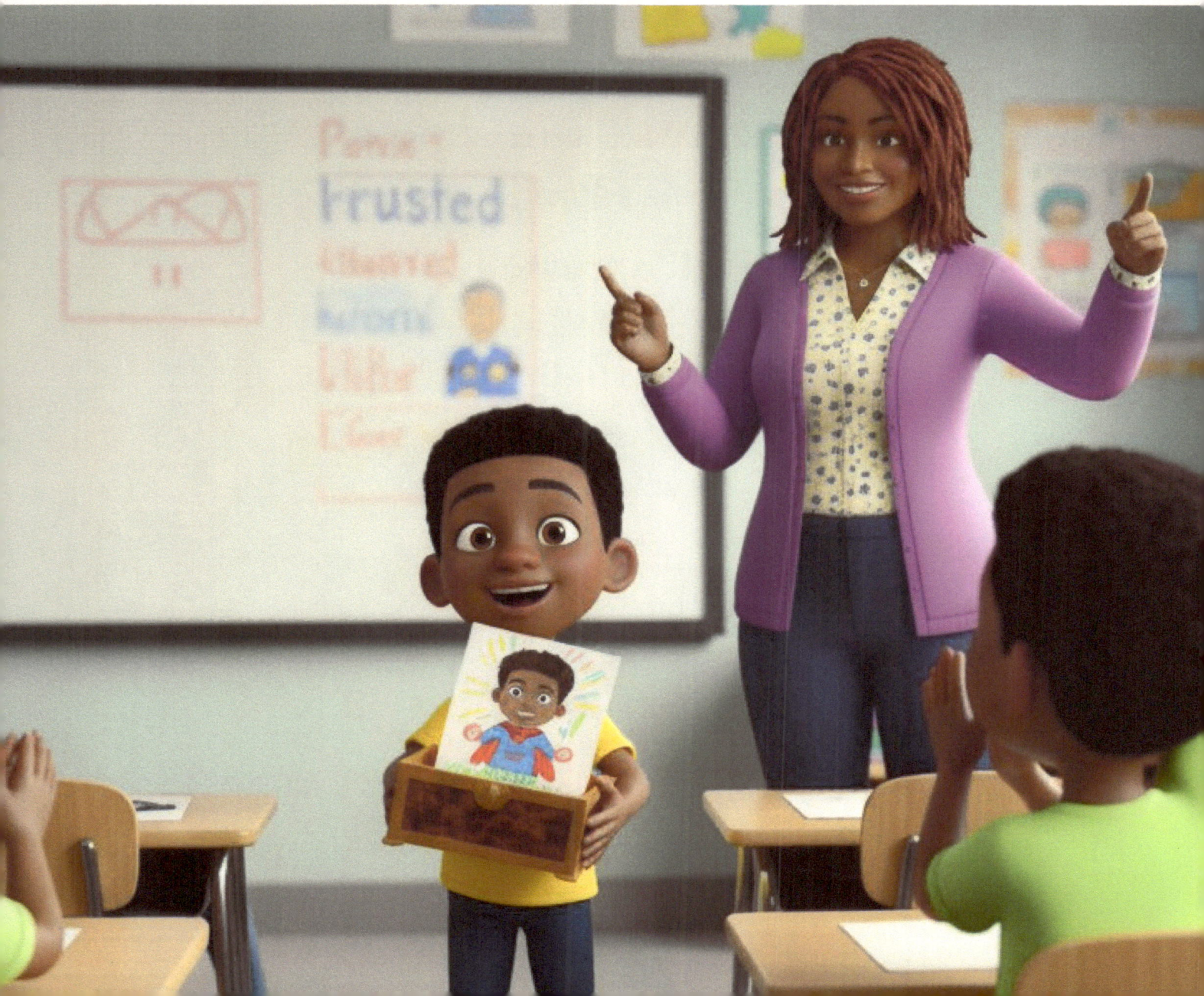

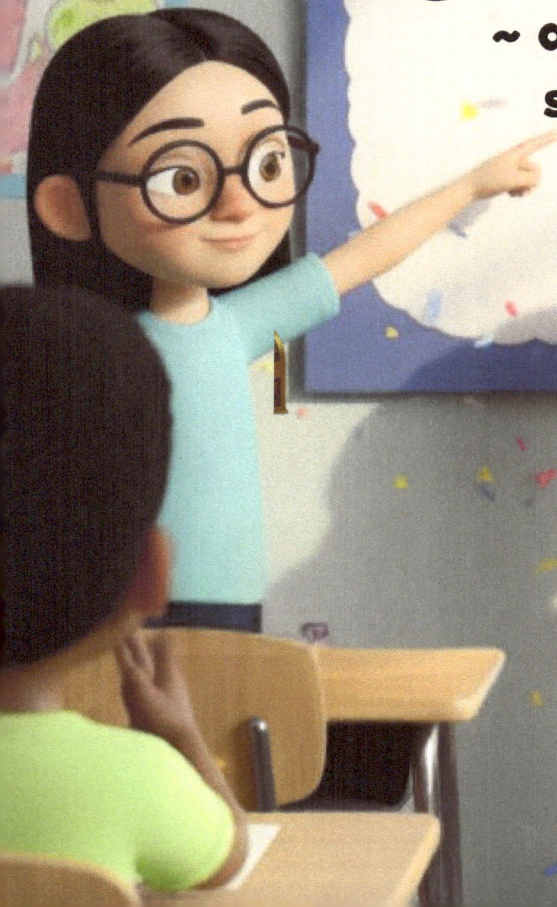

Parent & Educator Guide

Series: The Child Safety Book Package by Stacy Sylvain-Davis, M.S., M.Ed.
Age Group: Early Elementary (Ages 6–8)

Learning Objectives
• Identify and understand the difference between safe and unsafe secrets
• Recognize and trust "uh-oh" feelings that signal discomfort
• Practice assertive communication ("No, thank you," "I need to tell my mom")
• Reinforce the importance of telling a trusted adult—and continuing to tell until someone helps

Discussion Prompts
1. What kind of secrets are fun or happy?
2. What kind of secrets can make your tummy feel yucky or worried?
3. Who are three trusted adults you could talk to if something feels wrong?
4. How did Rome show bravery in the story?
5. What could you do if someone told you to keep a secret that felt unsafe?

Activities for Kids
1. Trusted Adult Map: Draw or list three adults who help you feel safe.
2. Safe vs. Unsafe Secrets Sort: Make two boxes - SAFE SECRETS and UNSAFE SECRETS - and sort examples.
3. Role-Play Practice: Act out safe and unsafe scenarios.
4. Journal Reflection: "When did I feel brave today?"

Tips for Parents & Educators:
• Validate feelings: It's okay to feel scared or unsure.
• Avoid shaming: It's never the child's fault.
• Use repetition: Review safety lessons often.
• Model communication: Share your own examples.
• Keep open dialogue: No secret is too big or small.

Key Takeaways for Kids:
1. Safe secrets make me feel happy inside. Unsafe secrets make me feel yucky.
2. My feelings help me know when something's wrong.
3. I can say **"No"** to anything that feels wrong.
4. I can tell a trusted adult - and keep telling until someone helps.

Let's Practice Together!

1. Safe or Unsafe Secret?
Read each one out loud together. Point to safe or unsafe.

- 🎁 Someone asks you to keep a secret about a surprise party.
- 😰 A grown-up tells you to keep something secret that makes your stomach feel yucky.
- 💐 Your class is making a surprise card for your teacher.
- 🤫 A neighbor says, "Don't tell your mom what happened."

2. My Body Feelings Check-In
Circle or point to the feeling:

- 🥰 *This feels happy and safe.*
- 🤔 *I'm not sure... something feels off.*
- 😰 *My stomach is twisting. This feels yucky.*

3. Who Are My Trusted Adults?
Write or draw the names of 3 people you can always tell.

1. _____
2. _____
3. _____

4. Practice Your Strong Voice
Repeat together:

"If a secret feels yucky, I can say 'No,' walk away, and tell a trusted adult."

I AM A SAFETY SUPERSTAR!

CERTIFICATE OF COURAGE

This certificate is proudly presented to:

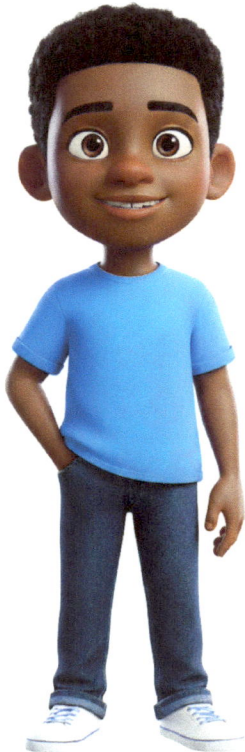

_____

for showing courage, kindness, and a strong voice ~
just like Rome!
You learned the difference between
safe secrets and unsafe secrets, and
you practiced speaking up to a trusted adult.
That makes you a true Safety Superstar!

Always remember:
"If a secret feels yucky, I can tell a trusted adult."

Date: _____

Signature: _____

(Parent, Teacher, or Safe Adult)

ABOUT THE AUTHOR

Stacy Sylvain-Davis, M.S., M.Ed., is an educator, author, and advocate dedicated to helping children feel safe, confident, and heard. As a survivor of childhood sexual abuse, she understands the power of a child's voice and the importance of early conversations about safety and boundaries.

With a background in education and years of experience supporting children and families, Stacy creates stories that teach emotional awareness, courage, and self-protection in simple, child-friendly ways.

When she's not writing, she enjoys time with her family and finding joy in life's everyday moments.

ABOUT THE SERIES

The Child Safety Book Package

The *Child Safety Book Collection* is a series of empowering, child-friendly stories designed to help children recognize unsafe situations, trust their feelings, and use their voices with confidence. Through gentle lessons and relatable characters, each book teaches important skills about boundaries, body safety, and speaking up.

Books in the Series:

- **JoJo Says, "No, Thank You!"**
  A story about recognizing unsafe touches and using your voice.

- **Rome and the Secret Box**
  A story about secrets, safe adults, and choosing courage.

- **She Learned Her Voice Could Keep Her Safe: TJ's Story**
  A story about trusting your feelings and asking for help.

This series is designed for families, classrooms, therapists, and ministries who want to protect and empower children with simple, meaningful tools for safety and confidence. Every child deserves to feel safe... and every voice matters.

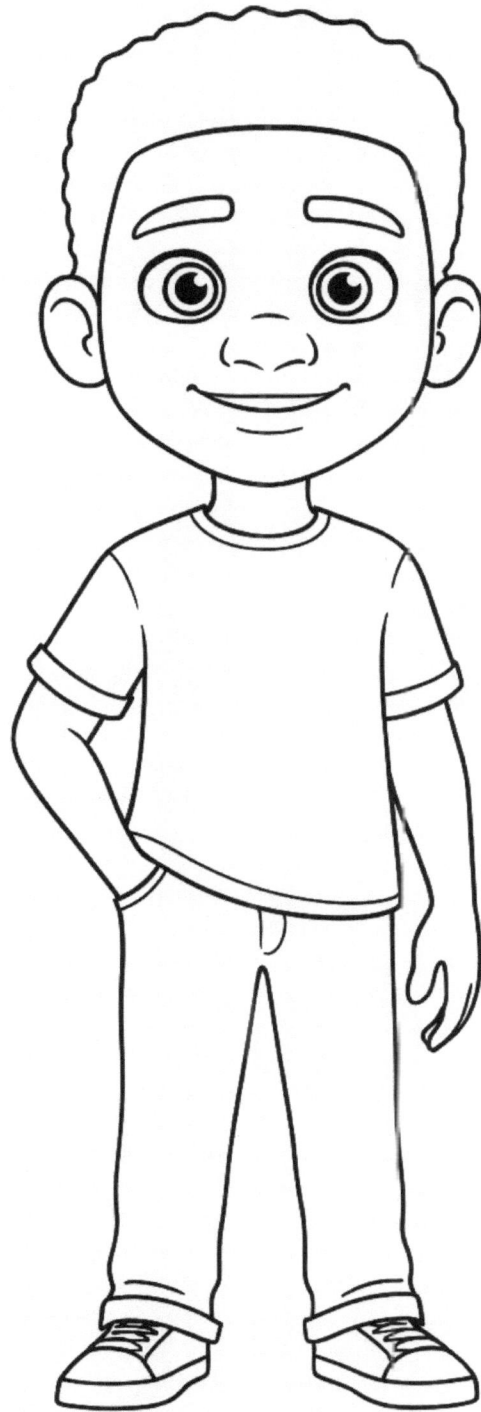

www.ingramcontent.com/pod-product-compliance
Lightning Source LLC
Chambersburg PA
CBHW060828270326
41931CB00002B/100